50 THINGS TO KNOW ABOUT KNOW ABOUT MAKING A DIFFERENCE

I0492593

Empowering you to impact your corner of the world

Marie Horne Wikle

Cover designed by: Ivana Stamenkovic
Cover Image: https://pixabay.com/photos/woman-girl-freedom-
happy-sun-591576/

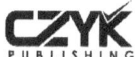

CZYK Publishing Since 2011.
CZYKPublishing.com
50 Things to Know

Lock Haven, PA
All rights reserved.
ISBN: 9798722396327

50 THINGS TO KNOW
BOOK SERIES
REVIEWS FROM READERS

I recently downloaded a couple of books from this series to read over the weekend thinking I would read just one or two. However, I so loved the books that I read all the six books I had downloaded in one go and ended up downloading a few more today. Written by different authors, the books offer practical advice on how you can perform or achieve certain goals in life, which in this case is how to have a better life.

The information is simple to digest and learn from, and is incredibly useful. There are also resources listed at the end of the book that you can use to get more information.

50 Things To Know To Have A Better Life: Self-Improvement Made Easy!

Author Dannii Cohen

This book is very helpful and provides simple tips on how to improve your everyday life. I found it to be useful in improving my overall attitude.

50 Things to Know For Your Mindfulness & Meditation Journey
Author Nina Edmondso

Quick read with 50 short and easy tips for what to think about before starting to homeschool.

50 Things to Know About Getting Started with Homeschool by
Author Amanda Walton

I really enjoyed the voice of the narrator, she speaks in a soothing tone. The book is a really great reminder of things we might have known we could do during stressful times, but forgot over the years.

Author Harmony Hawaii

There is so much waste in our society today. Everyone should be forced to read this book. I know I am passing it on to my family.

50 Things to Know to Downsize Your Life: How To Downsize, Organize, And Get Back to Basics

Author Lisa Rusczyk Ed. D.

Great book to get you motivated and understand why you may be losing motivation. Great for that person who wants to start getting healthy, or just for you when you need motivation while having an established workout routine.

50 Things To Know To Stick With A Workout: Motivational Tips To Start The New You Today

Author Sarah Hughes

50 THINGS TO KNOW ABOUT MAKING A DIFFERENCE

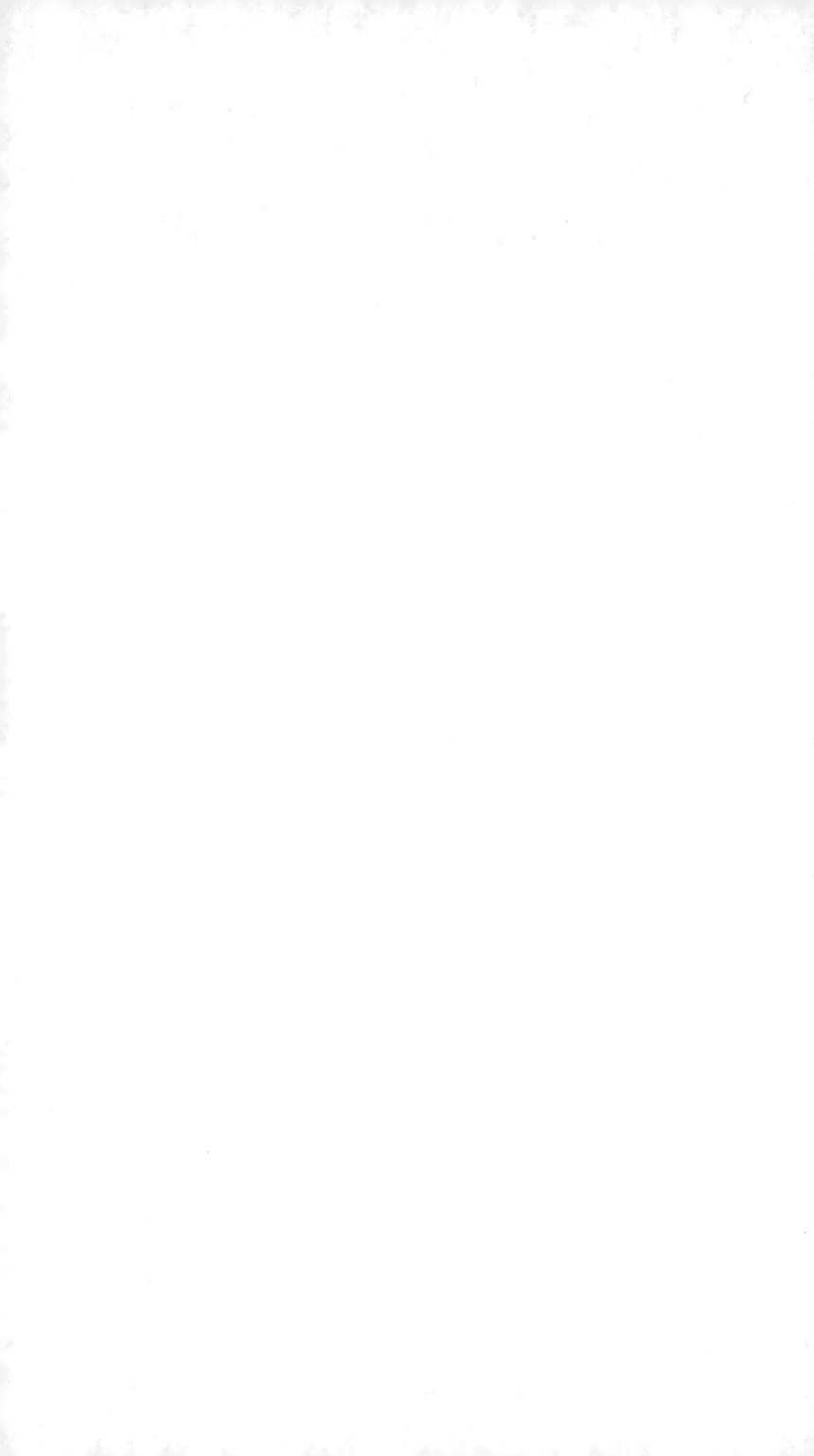

BOOK DESCRIPTION

Do you have a desire to make a difference in your corner of the world? Do you get discouraged when you can't give at the level your heart desires? Do you struggle with ideas of kindness and spreading joy to others that will fit into your budget?

If you answered yes to any of these questions then this book is for you!

50 Things to Know about Making a Difference by author Marie Horne Wikle offers an approach to making a difference each day without breaking the bank or allowing guilt to steal your joy of doing so. Most books on changing the world are full of ideas that only people with great financial resources or popular connections can actually achieve. Although there's nothing wrong with that, there are ways that anyone of any ages can have a positive impact on their world.

In these pages you'll discover the life changing effects that making a difference for others has on you personally. This book will help you with ideas, tips and suggestions that will enable you to focus on your own resources, reminding you that you are fully equipped to make a positive difference for the world around you.

By the time you finish this book, you will know how to make a difference without spending any money, you'll learn to look at the resources you have, your talents and gifts that allow you to naturally incorporate spreading joy to others in your day and you'll be reminded of the simplicity of kind words and a bright smile and the impact those items makes. So grab YOUR copy today. You'll be glad you did.

TABLE OF CONTENTS

DEDICATION

To every person of any age that has said "I wish I could make the world a better place for just one person"

ABOUT THE AUTHOR

Seeing through the eyes of compassion and understanding the heart that desires to have an impact, Marie encourages others to see the full potential of the everday, ordinary resources that is right within their reach.

Everyone needs to make a difference and with creative thinking and a unique look at the ordinary, she shows people all over the world just how easy it is to make a difference. Regardless of circumstances, everyone has it within themselves to make a difference. Marie has the desire to be the voice that reminds others that it can be done. Valuing the little things that make life big, seeing the extraordinary in the every day ordinary journey of life and choosing to cause joy while choosing joy is something that everyone can harness the power from within to accomplish.

Marie is currently working as a Salesforce Admin by day and Voice Over Artist by night (and weekends)

Where you find you on social media…

Twitter:

@spreadingJOY and @mariewikle

Facebook:

https://www.facebook.com/joyfullyyoursvoiceover

I am only one, but still I am one.
I cannot do everything, but still I
can do something; and because I
cannot do everything I will not
refuse to do something that I can do

– Edward Everett Hale

Everyone has the desire to make a difference in this world, to have a positive impact in their corner of the world and yet, they are discouraged before they even start.

The reason for this discouragement is because we feel like if we can't make a large, world changing difference, then why bother.

Many are discouraged because they can't donate thousands of dollars to their favorite charity. Others are discouraged because they can't pay off every layaway at their local store and then there's the group that can barely make ends meet and feel they have nothing left to offer.

This handbook will help you to move beyond these thoughts and feelings. Everyone everywhere has the ability right now to make a significant impact on this world. You are fully equipped with all you need to make a difference that will have limitless effects on those you help and encourage.

This book is filled with encouragement, motivation as well as ideas anyone of any age or financial status can quickly and easily implement.

1. GO BIG OR GO HOME

If you cannot feed a hundred
people, feed one.

– Mother Teresa

When thinking about the many various ways of making a difference, we often think of giving away $1,000,000 if we were to win the lottery. Or we dream of waltzing into a store and paying off every layaway at Christmas Time or purchasing a vehicle or home for someone in need, when in reality, we don't actually have to do things of that nature at all to have a life changing impact on others. All we have to do is consider our talents, resources and the opportunities that present themselves on a daily basis and we have all we need to be a positive force that this world needs. Get rid of all or nothing mindset when looking for ways to make a difference. Actively focus on something you can do for one person on one certain day and to it. Afterwards, do not allow guilt of not doing more steal your joy of helping someone. Think about how your kind words, meal for one person or box of diapers for a new mom would be the uplifting and encouraging boost that someone in your world needs.

2. KINDNESS MATTERS

*Believe with all your heart that
how you live your life makes a
difference.*

– Colin Brown

You don't have to pour money into charities to make
a difference, although it truly does help them. You
simply need to live a life of kindness, compassion and
positivity and you will absolutely have a positive
impact on everyone you encounter. Kindness is such
a rare trait these days. When people are easily
frustrated, allowing nothing but their anger to rage, be
the one who is patient, who displays kindness to
everyone and the one who allows positivity to flow
like a river of hope to a dry and thirsty world. Be kind
to the cashier who has endured 25 people telling them
that they are the worst. Be kind to your server who
has been told that the food is all wrong 5 times today.
Be kind to teachers who always hear how they are the
blame for their kids grades being low. Be kind to
your family who, just like you, are learning as they
go. It truly is that simple. Be kind.

3. THE POWER OF WORDS

*Sticks and stones will break my
bones by words will never hurt me.*

– Childhood Nursery Rhyme

I live in generation that said this little nursery
rhyme….quite a lot. The horrible truth is that YES,
words will hurt more than we can ever possibly
imagine. But, the opposite is also true. The power of
encouraging words, uplifting words, motivating
words is nothing short of miraculous! Many people
hold on to cards and handwritten notes they get so
that they can re-visit those powerful words. Many
people keep those notes of positivity handy as a
reminder of the good things that are sprinkled
throughout the day. Your words are powerful! Use
them often! Use them to encourage your family. Use
them to send cards or letters to those you do not get to
see very often. Use sticky notes and write something
nice on them for random people and stick to their
driver side windows as you walk past each car on
your way to the store. Stick a note with words of love
and encouragement in your child's bag for them to
find when they go to spend the night with a friend.
The possibilities here are endless! Use your words for
good!

4. MOMS HELPING HAND

No act of kindness, no matter
how small is ever wasted.

– Aesop

Do you know any single moms that could use a
helping hand or two? Do you know of a new mom
that could use a helping hand? Being a mom is a
tough job and sometimes that person that steps in at
just the right moment turns out to be quite the hero!
Maybe you know a new mom who could use a little
help with day to day items. Maybe you know a single
mom who could use an evening to herself but never
gets one because she can't afford a sitter? Think
about the things you excel at and how you can apply
those to help out moms in need. Can you bake extra
and give to a family? Can you send over a meal that
includes paper plates, cups and napkins, ensuring no
clean up is required? Can you purchase diapers and
wipes to help ease the financial strain these necessary
items cause? Look inward to your heart and abilities
and think of how you can use your current resources
to make a difference for moms in your corner of the
world. You don't know any single moms or new
moms you say? Or can't visit them due to health
issues? That's ok. Next time you are in the grocer
store, place a $10 bill in one of the diaper boxes that

have handles in it. Trust me! The mom will be beyond grateful! Making a difference where the recipient cannot thank you or even hug you will flood your own heart with great joy!

5. SMALL THINGS MAKE A BIG DIFFERENCE

Anyone who thinks that they are too small to make a difference has never tried to fall asleep with a mosquito in the room.

– The Dalai Lama

Everyone at any age is perfectly equipped to make a difference – right now! Think about the toddler that grabs a yellow weed from the grass and proudly brings it in as the most perfect gift. That weed is celebrated as the perfect glass vase is found and water put in. We know it will not survive the evening and it will most certainly be forgotten about in 3 seconds by the toddler but right now…it is the MOST perfect gift ever! Why? Because it was given from the heart, without concern about what it was or how much it cost. It was given because love demanded a gift be

11

found. It was given because beauty screamed "pick me, pick me" to the toddler. It was given because little things truly do matter. Stop focusing on what you cannot do and place your focus on your strengths. Do you have a bright smile? Use it! Do you have a rose garden or flower garden? Use it! Do you crochet, knit or make items that others will love? Do it! Are you a techy sort of person? Volunteer your time to a non profit. The point here is that NO ONE is too small to make a difference. You just haven't found what your heart is passionate about. Find it and do it!

6. KEEPING IT IN THE FAMILY

Never worry about numbers.
Help one person at a time, and
always start with the person nearest
you.

– Mother Teresa

Random acts of kindness and making a difference for people you do not know is such a fun thing to do. May I take this time to remind you that the same is true for your family! Yes, we are supposed to provide, encourage and show positivity to them but what about making it something special every once in a while? It doesn't have to be huge or expensive. Maybe let someone have their favorite meal with dessert one evening. Allow someone else to pick the movie and snacks for movie night. Provide turn down service to your family members by turning down their bed and leaving a small piece of chocolate on their pillow. You know what your family loves and what you can afford to do. Think about the resources you have and what you can easily implement today to start making a difference for those you love the most.

7. THE PURPOSE OF LIVING

*Regardless of whatever I do, I
know what my purpose is: to make
a difference in people's lives.*

– Tim Tebow

People everywhere are searching for THEIR purpose
in this life. Their reason for living, and learning how
to live life with meaning. While searching, please
please please – do not forget to seek out ways to
make a difference. What would life mean to be the
most successful person in the world and yet, never
use your gifts, talents or resources to help others.
Also, do not wait until you "have arrived" to start
making a difference for others either. If you wait until
then, you will miss out on many wonderful
opportunities to impact this world for good. While
you are climbing the ladder of success, encourage
those on their journey too. Leave notes of
encouragement for others to find. Someone help you
find your calling? Express gratitude to them.
Focusing on your current situation, current resources
be sure to scatter joy to others as you make your way
through the day.

8. ZERO EXPECTATIONS

*The way you treat people who
are in no position to help you,
further you, or benefit you – reveals
the true state of your heart.*

– Mandy Hale

I love seeing people helping people. I love hearing about someone who was helped out in a time of need. No matter what it is! It's always encouraging and uplifting. Please, when you are helping others, don't attach strings to it. Don't do it. Make a difference for others because you can. Support those in need because you understand what it's like. Help others with zero expectations in return about what they will do with your help or not do. If you give money to someone on the side of the road, just give it without worry about what they will do with it. If you donate clothes to a family in need, do it without expecting anything in return. Make a difference for others because you can, not because the event or action will be recorded and go viral. Remember, The best giving is often done in secret.

9. THE TIME IS NOW

*How wonderful it is that nobody
need wait a single moment before
starting to improve the world.*

– Anne Frank

Are you making a difference where you can, when
you can? If not, what are you waiting on? Don't wait
for "things" to get better. Look at your current
resources and see how you can help others. Does
writing come easy for you? Help women that are re-
entering the workforce for the first time in a long time
with their resume. Are you highly technical with
websites? Help those that are not. Are you good at
organizing events? Why not volunteer with your
favorite school or non-profit and help them with
events? The sky is literally the limit when it comes to
helping others and the time is now. Don't wait. Make
a difference for someone today!

10. MAKING A DIFFERENCE FOR OTHERS ALWAYS ENCOURAGES YOU

When you encourage others, you in the process are encouraged because you're making a commitment and difference in that person's life.

– Zig Ziglar

Have you ever thought to yourself "why should we even bother making a difference for others anyway?" If so, you are not alone. There are huge benefits when you are focused on others for a little bit of time. Not only does it help the one in need but your heart will also be encouraged. You will be flooded with great joy as you make a difference for others around you and even for those you don't even know. The next time you are struggling or are feeling down, seek out someone you can do something small for. Maybe it's giving a sincere compliment, or thanking a store manager for hiring great employees or even paying for the meal of the person behind you and watch how your heart is lifted and encouraged. You cannot sprinkle the confetti of joy on others without some of

17

it falling back down on yourself. This is why you should try and make a difference for ONE person a day. Just one.

11. WHAT IS YOUR LEGACY?

What we have done for ourselves alone dies with us; what we have done for others an the world remains and is immortal.

– Albert Pike

Don't be the one who leaves this world with nothing of yourself. Sprinkle seeds of happiness and joy everywhere you go. Leave others with a smile on their face and inspiration in their heart. When we remove the guilt and the huge giving level that everyone seems to only want to give on, then nothing is impossible to accomplish when you are making a difference for others. Can you meet all the needs of everyone you ever meet? Surely no one can do that. Can you leave everyone a little happier, a little more encouraged and lifted up? Yes! YES, everyone can absolutely do that! Stop focusing on what you can't do, what you wish you could do and what you would do if you won the lottery. START focusing on what you can do, those you can encourage and empower and do that!

12. STEP AWAY FROM THE COMFORT ZONE

We want to rise above the discouragement of high prices, the obstacle of dead ends and the disappointment of our comfort zone. We want to be the change that is so desperately needed.

– Marie Wikle

Does the thought of just waltzing up to someone and helping them make your heart beat out of control? Are you reading this book thinking "nope, I could never – ever do that in a million years?" I understand. I was painfully shy and super awkward in my teens and pre-teens. I wanted to vomit when doing book reports and I never (and I mean NEVER) went out of my way to speak to anyone I didn't know. I just didn't. Stepping out a little at a time enable me to be the person I am today. Someone prodded me to speak to one person I didn't know – just one. To my surprise, the world didn't end. They spoke back and life was still good. Making a difference for those you don't know can be a bit scary as you aren't sure how it will be received. I've had one person in my whole life respond negatively to my kindness. Just one. I didn't let it bother me. I kept reaching out and helping where I could. Doing one thing a day for someone is a small step that anyone can do. Even children. Take a little time to plan and you'll be super comfortable making a difference each and every day!

13. GET THE KIDS INVOLVED

How do you spell love? – Piglet
– You don't spell it, you feel it.

– Winnie the Pooh

Children are such creative master minds! Many kids see a need and they can come up with a solution giving the time and resources. There are apps to help kids not have to sit alone in the lunch room. There are kids that start non profits to help kids have books over the summer so they can keep reading and learning over the summer. There are kids who have sold lemonade and donated more than $50,000 to children and their families that are fighting cancer. Start now teaching your child to help others, without judgement or assumptions. Go to the dollar store and get a bunch of bears or stuffed dogs and then take to a nursing home to give away. Stop by McDonalds and get hot fudge sundaes and give to the road crew on a hot summer day. Wrap up some books your child no longer reads in pretty paper – mark it boy or girl and take to the park and leave in different places. Have fun making a difference while making amazing memories.

14. ENCOURAGEMENT TODAY BRINGS A BRIGHTER TOMORROW

Make a difference today for someone who's fighting for their tomorrow.

– Jim Kelly

You never know what people are going through. You can't know if their smile is genuine or a smile through pain. You don't know if the cashier snapped at you because her child is super sick and she has to work to just make ends meet or if the person sitting across from you who is angry at the world feels like the world is caving in on them. Be the difference for them today! Bring light into their world today! Give them hope for today so that they can get up again tomorrow and try again! Never assume you know what is going on with those you pass by. Be the one to bring positivity into their space!

15. KEEP IT SIMPLE

*Ultimately it's the simple things
that make a difference.*

– Chris Smalling

On this journey of making a difference for people, be sure to keep it simple. Don't over complicate it! You see a need that you can meet – do it. Let someone ahead of you in line, hold the door for someone. Buy a doze roses at the grocery store and give one to all the ladies as they exit the store. Making a difference for others doesn't require a lot of effort, just willingness.

16. MAKE IT A HABIT

*It's not what you do once in a
while, it's what you do day in and
day out that makes the difference.*

– Jenny Craig

We all try and better ourselves. We try to instill good
habits in our life. Have you thought of making a
difference for others a good habit for yourself? Every
opportunity you take to improve the world for
someone, you sprinkle joy on yourself too. Making a
difference for just one person a day will no doubt
inspire others around you to do the same. Your one
person now becomes two. Opportunities will arise
each day to encourage someone. You will not have to
look far. Leave an encouraging note in a book at the
library. Thank our first responders. Baby sit for free
for a single mom. Organize a book drive. Have a
family meal at the table and talk about current events.
It won't take long for this habit to leave an imprint of
love on your heart.

17. THE POWER OF A SINGLE SMILE

*A simple Smile. That's the start
of opening your heart and being
compassionate to others.*

– Dalai Lama

A smile breaks all language barriers. A simple smile will soften the toughest heart, heal a broken spirit and encourage even the most defeated of souls. Your Smile is that powerful too! Your smile may be the reassurance a young mom needs when her kids are not listening in the grocery store. Your smile will lift the spirits of the lonely widow woman who is missing her soul mate. Your smile will express gratitude to the cashier who has been yelled at 5 times today. Your smile will remind your family that they mean more than the world to you. Use the power of a simple smile to brighten the world of those you encounter each day!

18. BE AVAILABLE

Being available is more important than being desirable.

– Constance Chuks

Have you ever seen the tears in someone's eyes and the hurt in their heart and wish you had just the perfect words to say? Have you ever felt speechless in a moment when someone is experiencing great grief? That is normal and ok. The biggest thing you can do in that instance is to be there for them. Be available. Be by their side. Cry with them if you feel like crying. The beauty of this is that everyone can be available to those who are hurting.

19. DOUBLE RECIPES

*Food brings people together on
many different levels. It's
nourishment of the soul and body;
it's truly love.*

– Giada De Laurentiis

Those homemade cookies you are baking…. Make an
extra batch and take over to the local Firehouse for
those first responders. That homemade chili and
cornbread muffins you getting ready to whip up –
make extra for the elderly couple that lives 2 houses
down. You can do so many great things with the gift
of food if you simply double the recipe. No going out
of your way, no extra steps – just pure love.

20. SPEAK WITHOUT SAYING A WORD

Well done is better than well said.

– Benjamin Franklin

Making a difference is all about kindness, love and compassion towards others. Don't just think about doing it or wish you could do more. Use the ideas in this book to help generate other ideas based off your own resources. The possibilities are endless and the actions you take will scream out about the love you carry within. Can you mentor someone? Can you help fix the vehicle of someone in need? Can you run errands for those who cannot get out of their house for one reason or another? Be bold in your speech regardless if it's out loud or through your actions.

21. CHOOSE GRATITUDE

*Gratitude turns what we have
into enough.*

– Anonymous

We may never have all that we want or desire, but most of us will usually have more than what we actually need. Be thankful for it. For every little bit of it. Be thankful that you've been able to eat peanut butter sandwiches for the 3rd time this week and didn't go hungry. Be thankful that your care still runs after 15 years. Be thankful that the lights are on in your small, cramped home. Be thankful! Be thankful for the moon and stars that shimmer on the darkest night. Be thankful for the sun that radiates it's warmth for the world to enjoy. Be thankful for the kindness of others. Be thankful for that smile through the tears. Be thankful for the power to encourage others. Be thankful for the rainbow after the rain. Just be thankful! Today and everyday.

22. SHARE THE KIDS ARTWORK

*Children can see magic because
they look for it.*

– Christopher Moore

Do you have smaller children in your home that still love to draw and color? Share their work with family. There are so many apps that will allow you to take a photo and turn it into a post card and easily add an address and away it goes – mail of the happiest kind! That will be the highlight of the day for the special person you have chosen to receive it!

23. ZERO SPENDING

Everyone can be great, because
everyone can serve.

– Martin Luther King, Jr

People have asked me "how can I make a difference when I cannot even make ends meet?" Many people find themselves in this situation. Their finances are not the greatest but they still desire to make a difference in the world. There are so many ways to make a difference without spending a single cent. I'll share a few here:

• Donate blankets and clothing to organizations that will GIVE these things away

• Bake/make extra food

• Show sincere appreciation

• Leave an encouraging note on your mail box for your mail carrier

• Seek out a store manager and say good things about several of the employees

• Pick up trash when in public

• Pick flowers from your garden to give

24. SAY THANK YOU TO VETERANS

The meaning of life is to find
your gift. The purpose of life is to
give it away.

– Pablo Picasso

Say thank you to those who have served our country selflessly. Write some thank you cards in advance and keep them in your car so when you are at the store and you see a vehicle in the "veterans only" parking, you can leave it on their windshield. Or if you are in a restaurant and see an elderly gentleman with a hat on that represents what war he fought in, you can say thank you and hand him a card as well.

25. LEAVE REVIEWS

*Every charitable act is a
stepping stone towards heaven.*

– Henry Ward Beecher

Are there products that you love and use all the time?
Have the last few books you've read been simply
amazing? Why not take just a moment to leave a kind
review? It helps the author or owner of the product as
well as those that are looking to purchase. Kind words
truly are helpful!

26. ENCOURAGE YOUR SIGNIFICANT OTHER

One must know not just how to accept a gift, but with what grace to share it.

– Maya Angelou

Life is demanding and little things often get in the way and neglect the important people in our life. Encouragement is lasting and often doesn't cost a dime. Do little things for your significant other. Make and bring their coffee to them. Support their dreams. Have a lunch date or bring them their favorite dessert. Make time to laugh together on purpose. Little things like this have a lasting impact!

27. VOLUNTEER AT A SHELTER

Caring has the gift of making the
ordinary special.

– George R. Bach

There are so many types of shelters in any given city. Pick on and dive in. Make it a family affair. Help with food, clean up or organization. Wherever your talents are, use those to benefit this shelter and all of those that they help! Being here will remind you of the blessings you truly have while you are giving back and making a difference.

28. THANK YOUR CHILD'S TEACHER

*It is the supreme art of the
teacher to awaken joy In creative
expression and knowledge.*

– Albert Einstein

I love those that teach our children. They are brilliant,
kind and hold the future in our hands. They don't
seek wealth or fame, just helping our kids to be the
best they can be. Check on them. Thank them. Ask if
they need anything. Did you know most teachers have
a wish list on amazon of thing for their students. Or
they have a list of things written down that they
would love to have for their class. Ask. Or better yet,
instead of getting them another cup with teacher on it
(which they will love and adore) get them an amazon
gift card and a box of copy paper. They will be so
thrilled!

29. WHY MAKE A DIFFERENCE AT ALL?

*If there be any truer measure of
a man than by what he does, it must
be by what he gives.*

– Robert South

Most people reading this book will love the ideas and encouragement found in between each page. Yet, there will be others who simply as, why….why make a difference at all? That is a valid question. Why not just go on quietly living your life, doing the best you can to get by? In helping others, we truly do help ourselves. Our hearts are flooded with joy and overwhelming gratitude for the things we have. Other reasons are because doing a little is better than doing nothing. Doing something for someone that can never repay you IS it's own reward. There is true JOY in helping others. I make a difference for others because one day, I may be the one in need. I don't focus on being noticed, I focus on being useful.

30. CREATE CARE PACKS FOR HOMELESS

It's not about giving back if you're successful or a celebrity or how much money you have: It's about your responsibility as an adult to help others.

– Trisha Yearwood

It's ok if you don't like to give cash away to people. Many don't. You can create care packs and keep in your car for times you want to help those in need. Include things that don't go bad too quickly - like granola bars, single serve peanut butter and some crackers, bottle of water, new socks, instant coffee packs (many places gives free hot water) tea bags. Things that are small and useful. Take this one step further and fill your childs backpack that you no longer use with a few others things, like t-shirts, blanket and other hygiene items.

31. UNPLUG

Tension is who you think you should be. Relaxation is who you are.

– Chinese Proverb

While I love having the answer to anything at my fingertips, it is very important to actually unplug on purpose and just be. Doing this allows me to shift my focus and be more mindful of my surroundings. When you unplug and truly start to notice things around you, you'll be able to make a difference with your resources easier. You can put your talents to good use and start making plans for how you are going to be beams of light in the darkness.

32. IT'S MY PARTY AND I'LL GIVE IF I WANT TO

When you're in a position to have gotten so much, the gift at this point is giving back.

– Paul Stanley

Instead of receiving birthday gifts for yourself, ask others to make a donation to your favorite charity or purchase toys for places that make a difference at Christmas Time. Chances are, you have most all that you need. Use your special day to help those in need in a special way.

33. THE GOLDEN RULE

Do unto others as you'd have
them do to you.

– Golden Rule

One of the easiest ways to make a difference for others is treating others the way you want to be treated. Think about how you react to situations you face. If you would not want someone reacting that way to you, change the way you react. I try and take this even a step further and treat people better than I expect to be treated. It's noticed and it truly does make a difference.

34. DELIVER MEALS

No one is useless in this world who lightens the burdens of another.

– Charles Dickens

There are many people who are home bound for one reason or another. If you know of the elderly or someone who is sick and cannot get out, deliver meals for them. Pick up essential items for them. Bring them something fun, cute and adorable to help them to smile more. Everyone can make a difference for someone; you simply need to be aware of the opportunities that surround you.

35. BE AWARE

You can have everything you
want in life if you just help enough
people get what they want in life.

– Zig Ziglar

As you can see by now making a difference isn't difficult or impossible. It's simply taking advantage of the opportunities that present themselves to you, or actively planning ways in which you can make a difference sometime during the day. Be aware of your surroundings. Notice the little things going on. Those are the times that the little acts of joy you sprinkle into someone else's life will matter the most and have the deepest impact.

36. LOOK BEHIND YOU

Those who are the happiest are
those who do the most for others.

– Booker T. Washington

I love hearing from others who say someone ahead of them in line bought their coffee or even their order of food for them. If you've never had this happen to you, it truly is an amazing thing! Why not try it. If you are in a line for coffee or fast food place, ask to pay for the order for the person behind you. It will lift your spirits, the person serving at the window will be able to pass the wonderful gift along and the person receiving the surprise of their order being covered will float through their day.

37. PROVIDE WARMTH

*Giving back involves a certain
amount of giving up.*

– Colin Powell

Go through your closets and get some of the blankets
that you no longer use for those in need. This can be
any time of the year. People struggle for many
reasons but having the comforts of a warm blanket
truly can warm the soul.

38. TIP EXTRA

*To do more for the world than
the world does for you, that is
success.*

– Henry Ford

You'd be surprised how many people simply do not tip when going out to eat. For many people, tipping well is more than the service they receive, it's gratitude for not having to mess up the kitchen to cook. It's gratitude for having time to simply enjoy a meal with nothing to do afterwards. Tipping is gratitude. When we eat out at breakfast we typically tip $10 because we know that the servers receive 15% of 7 bucks and that is not a lot. Try tipping extra at any meal. Not just the standard 15%. Also – leave a note on your ticket for your server and brighten their day a little more.

39. SEND A CARE PACKAGE FOR NO REASON

*To ease another's heartache is
to forget one's own.*

– Abraham Lincoln

Need some extra sunshine in your world? Send some sunshine to someone else. No special reason is needed. Doing it just because is such a fun thing. A quick search on Pinterest for sending a box of sunshine will reveal already done for you tags, templates and suggestions of all things yellow to include in your box. The same is true for every color of the rainbow! Imagine how you would feel if you opened a box of "Sunshine." Now…. Go, get some sunshine for someone else!

40. MONTHLY NO CHORE DAY

Life is not a race, but a journey
to be savored each step of the way.

– Brian Dyson

You have a few short years with your family. Yes, I get that you want your home clean and you work hard all week and need Saturdays to catch up. Once in a while, monthly even, take time to have a no chore day. Plan on fun this day. Plan ahead and get the chores done a little early if you must. Take a day to play, relax, read, do crafts together or do nothing together. Thing is, do something different. Let someone else plan it. You have 12 wonderful months to take just one day to simply be together! Make is special!

41. ADOPT A GRANDPARENT

*Since you get more joy out of
giving joy to others, you should put
a good deal of thought into the
happiness that you are able to give.*

– Eleanor Roosevelt

We truly do get more joy in making a difference than
any other way in life. This is why it's so important to
help the elderly. Do you know some elderly that live
in your neighborhood? A Senior Living Center near
by? Go and adopt grandparents from there. Send them
cards, notes and stickers. Take stuffed animals and
find out what kind of puzzle books they love. Get
large print so they can see it easier.

42. DELIGHTFUL SNAIL MAIL

*In our throwaway era of quick
phone calls, faxes and email, it's all
too easy never to find the time to
write letters. That's a great pity for
historians and the rest of us.*

– Nancy Reagan

With all the bills and junkmail that gets tossed into
our mail boxes, the handwritten note inside a card is
such a delight! Even children love getting mail!
Especially once they start to read and can see their
own name imprinted on the envelope. Sending snail
mail truly does make a difference! People can enjoy it
over and over again. It floods their heart and yours
with great joy. Do you know calligraphy? Lucky you!
Doll up the outside or the inside even. Sending cards
and letters in the mail is like sending a warm hug!
Who do you need to send a hug to today?

43. JAR OF MEMORIES

*Memory is the diary we all carry
about with us.*

– Oscar Wilde

Grab a pretty jar or a plain jar and pretty it up. Cut strips of paper and put in special memories right after they happen. We always think we will remember this forever, but truth is, we don't. Also – individualize the jar and sneak in some "I like you because….." or "I love you because…." To the person that owns the jar. What a wonderful surprise this will be for them when they take the time to go through their memories. Be sure to jot down the date on the slip of paper and the age of the person.

44. SLOW DOWN

*The hurrier I go, the behinder I
get.*

– Lewis Carroll

We've all been there. When we are rushed and in a
hurry it seems like every thing that can go wrong,
will. If it can bother you, it will. If it can get on your
last nerve….it will. Stop rushing around like the sky
is falling and slow things down a bit. Take a nice long
deep breath or 4 and then begin again with specifics
in mind. Not everything has to be done today, but
things that are done today should be done well. Slow
down.

45. END WITH POSITIVITY

You're off to great places, today
is your day. Your mountain is
waiting, so get on your way.

– Dr Seuss

I realize that not everything or everyday can end on a positive note, but it is certainly worth the effort to try. Leave with a smile, say I love you before leaving your loved ones. End every thing that you can on a positive note. Negativity tries to drown out the good in each day. Getting yourself in the habit of ending things on a positive note will help bring positivity back to center stage.

46. PACKS OF JOY FOR KIDS

*Little things make a big
difference.*

– Yogi Berra

Getting your kids involved in making a difference is
as easy as a trip to the dollar store. Get some cello
bags, stickers, stamps and other little things. When
you get home, put on some fun music and lay
everything out in groups and assemble your bags.
Have your child draw smiley faces or hearts or even
flowers on some paper that you've cut into 4 squares
and put the word smile on it. Take them to a local
women's shelter or even go back to the dollar store
and allow your child to hand them out to kids that are
with their parents. Another way to give them out is to
walk through a McDonald's or other fast food place
just to give them away and then treat your child to a
hot fudge Sunday or ice cream cone. Allow them to
feel how making a difference for others floods their
world with joy.

47. SPECIAL DELIVERY

*We can do no great things, only
small things with great love.*

– Mother Teresa

Deliver something special to someone you love. It
could be pizza to the guy in your world, comic books
to the fan that still loves these. It could be a box of
books for the avid reader in your world. It could be
coffee with various creamers for the coffee lover in
your world. Think about the things that those who are
close to you truly love and adore. Do something
different and special to remind those close to you that
they are special too.

48. STICKY NOTE OF ENCOURAGEMENT

No matter what anybody tells you, words and ideas can change the world.

– John Keating

Making a difference is as easy as purchasing a sticky note pad and writing YOU MATTER on each one of them and leaving them in random places. Leave them on windshields or car windows. Leave them on bathroom mirrors. Leave them in magazines or books. Push them through the handles on the larger diaper packs. You can draw a smiley face or heart or flower or any of your favorite doodles. People are discouraged, people feel down and useless. Seeing this message may be what that person needs on that day to simply take the next step. This will have a limitless effect that you will never know the extent of it's reach. You can fill out your stick notes while watching tv or waiting in line. Have fun encouraging others and making a difference!

49. WAYS TO MAKE A DIFFERENCE

*The secret of change is to focus
all your energy, not on fighting the
old, but on building the new.*

– Socrates

This book has been full of tips and ideas to show you just how easy it is to make a difference right where you are with what you have AND without feeling guilty. You can do this! You were built to help others. Before we end this book, I wanted to jot down a few ideas that will help you even more. Again, you may not be able to do everything in this book, but you can think about your talents and resources and start right there. These ideas are meant to bring about ideas that you can do.

• Teach a child to read

• Teach an older person how to use their smart phone and apps

• Plant flowers in public areas

• Volunteer for Special Olympics

• Help the elderly around the inside and outside of their home

- Pick up trash in public spaces

- Help build a home for Habitat for Humanity

- Build a book box in a low income area and make sure it always has books

- Listen to really hear

- Around Christmas, Go to the Post Office and ask for some "Santa Letters" and be Santa

50. CELEBRATE LIFE

Once you start celebrating the little victories in life, you will realize just how infinite they truly are.

– Alicia Emamdee

These two simple words are so powerful. Celebrate Life! Celebrate waking up, celebrate delicious coffee, tea or whatever it is you start your day with. Celebrate the season, the day, the rain or sun. Celebrate! Can you imagine what a happier world we would be living in if we celebrated each and every day? Start today and celebrate and watch how your heart soars and overflows with great joy, gratitude and happiness!

OTHER RESOURCES:

For ideas to make a difference each day, check out the book Spreading Joy Daily
https://amzn.to/2Ujz0wd

For ideas to make a difference without spending a single penny visit - http://www.spreading-joy.org/site/50-ways-to-make-a-difference-without-spending-a-penny/ or here
https://youtu.be/fR6dqjnZjnQ

Get started with the 30 Day Challenge – You'll get one email a day with 3 ideas right in your in box:
http://www.spreading-joy.org/site/30-days-of-spreading-joy/

READ OTHER
50 THINGS TO KNOW
BOOKS

50 Things to Know About Coping With Stress: By A
   Mental Health Specialist by Kimberly L.
   Brownridge

50 Things to Know About Being a Zookeeper: Life of
   a Zookeeper by Stephanie Fowlie

50 Things to Know About Becoming a Doctor: The
   Journey from Medical School of the Medical
   Profession by Tong Liu MD

50 Things to Know About Knitting: Knit, Purl, Tricks
   & Shortcuts by Christina Fanelli

50 Things to Know

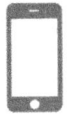

Stay up to date with new releases on Amazon:

https://amzn.to/2VPNGr7

CZYKPublishing.com

50 Things to Know

We'd love to hear what you think about our content! Please leave your honest review of this book on Amazon and Goodreads. We appreciate your positive and constructive feedback. Thank you.